Five Ways to Achieve Health Harmony and Happiness In 2015

J. Guinan Stevens and C.L. Carmen

DEDICATION

Our Heartfelt Thanks To Dr. and Mrs. Stevens

CONTENTS

YES YOU CAN Get on the PROGRAM!!!!!

Health , happiness and abundance are your birthright claim them!

All you have to do is go along this journey with us and let us show you how you can have everything that you desire.

There is one catch and it is We can't do it for you. No one else can its all up to you and you alone. Right now in this moment We are asking you to make a choice

Do you want o live, love and thrive or do you want to die with so many regrets? Think about it... really think about it.

The alternative to that option is to learn to love yourself for who and what you are in the present moment. Not who you were, or who you want to be. Learn to love the you that is right now.

1 **THE PROGRAM:A BRIEF OVERVIEW**

      This program is an economical no nonsense way of getting healthy, happy, and prosperous in all aspects of your life. The program consists of five pillars of protection for your mind, immune system, and your spirit. Each pillar is simple, it often boils down to being more mindful of your choices when it comes to that aspect of your life; for example always use what you have and replace the staples of your life with the best ingredients that you are able to. Try not to waste and make choices that are wise instead of based on impulses. That being said let us delve into the pillars themselves.

      The first Pillar of protection has to to with the mind. The first thing that has to change in your life is your mental perception. Negativity blocks us, not just emotionally but physically and spiritually as well. The first step in becoming a healthy person is to change your paradigm. Once the mind starts to change the body will follow. You will find yourself not wanting to harm yourself or anyone else. Naturally as you become more mindful you will find that your eating habits will start to change. Which leads us to the second pillar of the program... Diet. The old saying, "*you are what you eat from your head down to your feet,*" is true: if you want to be a healthy super strong person you must ingest super foods. It is exactly like Popeye and his spinach. Which leads us to the third pillar... exercise. A positive mind coupled with a properly nourished body gives you the energy to build a body that reflects all the change happening on the inside. We are not talking about running marathons, unless that is your dream. We are talking about simple life changes, about getting up and active. Every little bit helps. Once your mind is working positively, you are being mindful of what you eat, and you start and you start strengthening your body through exercise you are ready for the fourth pillar of the program... Supplementation.

Supplementation is very important these days. Eat all the calories you like, we doubt that you will get all the vitamins that your body needs to function properly. This pillar requires the use of daily vitamin supplements to strengthen you on a cellular level. Which bring us to the fifth pillar of the program....the Oxygen Cleanse. You are going to cleanse your body of all past infections while strengthening your immune and cardiovascular system. This is all done with an affordable, safe easy to do home therapy. You will have the power of oxygen working for you. This brings us to the sixth pillar of the program. Which is lacto fermentation. Now that you are thinking positively, eating mindfully, living an active lifestyle, supplementing your diet, and purifying your entire system it is time to take your diet to the next level. This is fermentation. It is easy, cost effective, preserves food, and is just plain delicious. Not to mention the fact that it helps to supercharge your immune system. The seventh pillar of the program is to cleanse the sinus and oral cavities. These are the places where we are most likely to catch bugs and viruses: ears, nose, throat, mouth and eyes. So it is imperative to have this system functioning at peak performance. This brings us to the Eighth and final pillar of the program.... Kvass. Kvass is the second of our miracle elixirs, the first being the Oxygen Cleanse. Beet Kvass is simple to make and incredibly nourishing. Now that you know what you are in for its time to take a more in depth look at each of the pillars independently. This program is uncomplicated, if we can do this anyone can. Failure is not trying in the first place. Your journey to absolute health and resistance to disease begins now.

2. __THE MIND__

Our brain is our best friend and our worst enemy. Like the yin-yang, it must be in balance. To attain that balance it must be clean, so that clarity and ease can be attained. With ease comes health and happiness. We must banish the dis-ease from our minds to ensure a clear pathway to ultimate health. In order to do this you must empty your mind of all negativity past and present. You must learn to forgive yourself for your perceived past mistakes and learn to truly forgive others. You cannot spend anytime on a,"what if,";or an, "I should have,"; or even a, " I cannot believe that they did that to me." The past is gone and there is nothing that you can do to bring it back, nothing at all. Woulda, coulda, shouldas are not allowed. Let it all go resolutely. Do it for real! Forgive yourself and stop punishing yourself. You deserve to live and be the healthiest you that you can be. It is okay to be happy with who you are and what your circumstances are. Stop comparing yourself to everyone else. The only marker for your yardstick is you. How much do you want to grow? You at this moment are the best you that you can be. You also have the opportunity at this very moment to become the person of your dreams. You can become whatever or whomever you desire starting right now. As you forgive others that have hurt, belittled, or done you wrong, no matter how bad, you will start to build spiritual strength. As you forgive these people and release them from your thoughts you will be getting rid of massive amounts of oppressive negativity. This process is long and on going. Your subconscious mind has been feeding on negativity in connection with these people and events for a long time. So you have to accept that it is going to take a sustained effort on your part. You cannot change negative thought patterns overnight or even in a week. It requires commitment to flood your mind with positive thoughts of forgiveness toward others and most importantly yourself. We are our own worst critics, and for most of us no one is harder on us than ourselves. We have experienced all the offenses, rejections, disappointments, injuries, and worst of all failures. We have been there and been first hand witnesses to all our mistakes, failures, and bad decisions. The worst of all these is when we let ourselves down, when we lie to ourselves, and injure ourselves both mentally and physically. The human condition is to have all these things and worse thrown at you. Life is very hard. Interacting with people professionally and socially is very difficult. Living in our own skins and interacting with ourselves can be arduous. As humans we are naturally judgmental. We judge things. Which piece of fruit is better. We also judge other people and ourselves, often negatively. It is just a natural tendency in today's society to have a negative spin on everything. To be super healthy we need to flood our minds with loving thoughts of forgiveness and good will towards others and most importantly ourselves. The old saying forgive and forget is more challenging to do than it sounds. We have all experienced people being extremely awful and doing horrible things to us, they inflict injuries that do not go away overnight. But slowly over time you will gain the power to let it all go and when you do, what a glorious happy day it will be. Positive thought is a very powerful thing. The problem is that society overwhelms us with negative imagery and thoughts through our media and entertainment. When negative thoughts rule the mind it is dis-eased, not at ease. When you consciously input positive, loving thoughts of forgiveness you are slowly putting your mind at ease and entering a healthy state. Once you have begun the process of forgiveness it is time to take it to the next level. You have to release all pettiness and jealousy from your life. It is by no means easy, but the rewards are definitely worth the effort. Release the negative thoughts and comparisons to others and you will reap the benefits of a healthy mind that will help you attain whatever goals you desire in life. Now that we are feeding healthy positive thoughts into our minds we are ready to move to the last step of mind for our purpose. That is gratitude. Gratitude is one of the most powerful emotions that we experience in life. It is right up there with love. It is interesting to note that negative hurtful emotions such as anger and hate are far easier to produce than the higher more powerful emotions of love and forgiveness. The more we can be grateful and experience that emotion, the stronger our mind and spirit becomes. As humans we always look at what we do not have. We focus on our wants, desires and what we lack. This floods our psyches with negativity and we become focused on lack, want, and what we do not have. As our conscious thoughts are feeding this lack into our subconscious, we are actually doing ourselves great harm. Because our subconscious does not judge it just listens and reacts. If you give it negative thoughts of what you lack that is exactly what your subconscious will reproduce in your life and experiences in this world. If you consciously input thoughts of love, forgiveness,empathy, and gratitude(all the highest of emotions), that is exactly what your subconscious will manifest in your life and experiences. As you gain power over your own thoughts and transform your mind into a powerhouse of positivity you will be amazed to see how quick the body follows. A healthy mind and body can fight off virus, bacteria and toxins. A healthy mind and body is ready to survive even the worst circumstances. There are many ways to achieve loving, positive, forgiving, grateful thoughts. Here are some traditional and not so traditional methods that can help get your mind in a healthy state.

The most traditional method is through meditation, reflection, and actually placing affirmative thoughts in your mind. This is easy, completely free, and does not take that much time. The result is not instant, it is cumulative. The more you focus on positivity, the more you remove negativity and sickness from your mind. It is an ongoing pursuit that takes commitment. A few brief affirmations at the end of this chapter will be included if this is one of the courses you pursue.

Another traditional method to getting rid of negativity would be therapy, or psychiatric care. Psychiatrists and therapists have been helping people put there mind at ease for generations. I would
caution however against the prescription of psychoactive drugs. These defeat the whole purpose of this book. We are trying to make you healthy on a cellular level so that you are highly resistant to viral infection, not put you on a new drug that could possibly compromise your immune system and overall health. If you are already on medication you can do the program, but check with your doctor first. However there are many psychiatrists and therapists who do not rely on drugs to solve problems. They actually work through your problems and issues. Therapy can be a wonderful and freeing process that can definitely put your mind at ease. There are only two downsides. Therapy can be a very

long and drawn out process. Therapy also is probably the most expensive option.

Another option is Hypnotherapy. Whether with an actual hypnotherapist or from a download hypnotherapy is very effective. When you see a hypnotherapist they make a recording of your session that you can listen to while relaxing every day. You can also download or buy recordings to be hypnotized at your leisure. Hypnotherapists can be quite expensive, but highly effective over time. Downloads and recordings are very affordable and in our opinion just as effective. hypnotherapy can be affordable, but it also takes a long term commitment to get full results. What we have found to be the most cost effective and gratifying are subliminals,binaural beats, and audio entrainment. By simply going onto youtube.com and performing a simple search of the above key words you will open up a world of possibilities. You will have a lot of choices but stay focused and listen to the ones that are going to help you with your goal of getting your mind in order. We have found that they are very effective to listen during our daily commute to and from work on the subway. Never ever listen to binaural beats, hypnosis, or do any sort of entrainment while driving or operating any sort of motor vehicle. Those are a couple of options to help cleanse your mind of negativity and strengthen your brain and overall health. As your mind becomes positively charged it will take a natural interest in your overall health. The next steps in the process will happen almost automatically.

We have included a few positive affirmations which will help accelerate the process. We take a spiritually neutral tone with with these affirmations. We encourage you to personalize them for yourself. They can be changed to fit your personal religious or spiritual beliefs. The main thing is that you believe in something higher than yourself even if it is the Laws of Physics, or your subconscious.

Affirmation of forgiveness:

I know that the power of the universe flows through me as forgiveness. I forgive all those that have hurt me, done me wrong, or led me astray. I forgive you all and release you to the universe. I forgive anyone who has offended me today. I forgive myself for the negative thoughts and actions that I havehad, and for any negative or hurtful thoughts that I have had today. I firmly resolve to have positive, constructive
thoughts of love. My thoughts are always onwards and upwards.

Affirmation of gratitude:
I know that the power of the universe flows through me as gratitude. I am grateful for all the blessings that the universe has bestowed upon me. I am grateful for my health, my family, my friends, my career, and even my wonderful possessions. I am so lucky for everything I have. I am thankful for all the wonderful blessings and treasures that the universe is going to bestow upon me. I am truly thankful that all my goals are being achieved successfully. Thank you very much.

Affirmation of health:

I know that the power of the universe flows through me as universal healing power. Universal healing power flows through me eliminating everything unlike itself. I am healing and being regenerated on a cellular level. My body is in perfect health and immune to all infection, viruses, bacteria, toxins and parasites. I give thanks for my perfect health. Thank you.

Affirmation for universal well being:

I know that I am the physical expression of the power of the universe. I know that universal power manifests itself within in me as health, happiness, abundance, joy and love.

Repeat these affirmations in comfort and silence two to three times per day and you will have amazing results within a week or two. Get your mind under control, you are in charge of it. Make it manifest what you truly want in your life. When you control your thoughts everything else in life seems to fall into place. As your brain becomes healthier you will find yourself making better decisions automatically, which then leads us to our second pillar.

3 GET YOUR BODY RIGHT

Diet is one of the most important things you can change to strengthen your immune system. This is not a book about weight loss. This is a book about making small changes in your life immediately that will cumulatively transform your life to complete health happiness and abundance throughout the course of the year.

Diet is very hard for most people. We either do not care about it and let ourselves go, or we go to the other extreme and over control our diets and often develop illnesses of the mind and body. For the purpose of this book we want you to make a mindful effort to make healthy choices in your diet. We want you to be well nourished and happy. In our current world civilization and world economic markets we have let the genie out of the bottle when it comes to food. In many countries in the world, the United States for example, we have access to affordable empty calories. If you have a dollar in your pocket you can go to McDonald's get a Mcdouble, and get a penny back! That is 390 calories right there. If you have another buck in your pocket they have some sort of soda deal, where you can get as many refills as you want. Soda is cheap access to calories. We have been there, seen it, and unfortunately done it many times in the past. The most affordable calories in the United States are the unhealthiest. They are all the ones that you can get coupons for. If you are poor in the U.S. the least healthy food is exactly what you have access to because it is the most affordable. Now what if you are not poor and you invest in the best brands and buy your foods from high end grocery stores? We do not believe that the rich are in a better position when it comes to healthy diets. In the U.S. we currently are experiencing a food disaster. Our diets as a whole are terrible. We are the most obese nation in the world. According to the Monday, September 8, 2014 issue of Time Magazine by 2048 100% of Americans will be obese. Diabetes, heart disease, and obesity are just a few of the ailments that are growing rampantly. In the U.S. we are literally eating ourselves to death. If your diet is compromised, your immune system is also at risk. We do not expect you to transform your whole diet over night, but we do expect you to be conscious of what you eat. We also expect you to try to make healthier choices from this point forward.

When you are first confronting your diet do not throw away what is in your cabinet or your fridge. Read the label before you prepare it, look at the portion size and adhere to it. The first step in controlling your diet is to actually know what you are eating and how much of your caloric intake for the day you are using up. We found a really great free app that we use religiously it is called *My Fitness Pal.* It tabulates everything for you and is quite easy to use. It has become an invaluable tool. Eat what you have until it is gone and then replace it with higher quality nutrient rich foods. We found ourselves craving lots of carbohydrates in the beginning. That precipitated feelings of deprivation, which allowed us to rationalize the buying of chips and gobbling them up. What we learned was do not deprive yourself of anything, just pay attention to the portion size. If you want chips eat them but do it responsibly.

Your body needs to be tamed just like your mind. When we spend a lifetime filling our bodies with caffeine, sugars, empty carbohydrates, and fat, we have to then ease it off gently. If you try to quit cold turkey you are asking for failure. Take your time and gently come off of the over processed foods. Always remember to restock with natural or organic alternatives. Start cooking quality nourishing simple meals. You can do it.

We used to be the household that scoured the weekly grocery circulars looking for the best deals on Sodas that we could find. Three twelve packs for $ 8.00 was brilliant, Five for $10.00 was even better. We felt elated when we looked in our fridge, and it was stocked with our weekly haul and then one day it just happened. Suddenly the hard core Cola was being swapped out for Diet versions. It was a natural transition. It happened and we did not fight it. Listen to your body when it tells you that it is okay to change. Over time we stopped going to the grocery store every week looking for the best soda deal because we had gobs of it at home in the fridge unopened. Hmm… something was going on and then we realized that we did not need the soda anymore. Naturally we started replacing soda with water. One day we brewed some green tea. We put it in a pitcher,stuck it in the fridge, and to our surprise it was delicious. Your body will automatically adjust itself to your healthier eating habits. We are all addicted to the additives in our food. It is up to us as adults to break the cycle of addiction and to teach our children how to eat responsibly. There is an old saying," *eat to live don't live to eat.*"We are asking everyone that lives in the world to embrace that mantra.

Medical science can do a plethora of things, but you only get one body. One temple to worship the benevolent God that you are becoming. Your mind is becoming more settled and your body is being nurtured from the inside. You should be feeling much more in control of everything. That is because you are freeing yourself from the shackles of negativity, the chains that bound you to eat from a place of emotional need. Which was a place of illusionary comfort rather than of sustenance. Stick with it, you are going to feel exceptional.

Become as healthy as you can no matter what your economic circumstances are. If vegetables are on sale purchase as many as you can. It is quite simple to make your own frozen veggies. Simply blanche (dip them for a few moments in boiling water), then remove the vegetables from the water, and place in a large bowl to cool. When you can handle them without burning yourself put standard servings into a freezer bag, remove all the air and put in the freezer. If you have enough variety make mixes just like they do in the store, let your imagination loose and have fun. If you can afford to buy a cry o-vac machine do it. If you want to eat red meat do it by all means. You should make the decision to eat less but of a higher quality and remember portion size. Save your colon some work, it is essential for the digestive system. It is in your digestive track that good health must flourish in order for you to live in ultimate health.

We must also pay attention to kitchen safety because hopefully you are spending more time in it. Be sure that all of your knives are sharp, a dull knife is an accident waiting to happen. It is vital that all of your surfaces are clean and that you wash all of your fruits vegetables and meats. Parasites and bacteria are not welcome in our healing bodies. At this point you have begun to work on the mind and the energy that fuels your body. Now it is time to burn some of that fuel. So far we are improving the thoughts that we are putting into our minds, and what we are nourishing ourselves with. Addressing these two things alone will greatly increase your health and immunity. Now it is time to step up to the next level with exercise. We do not expect you to rush out the door and join the most expensive gym. We do not expect you to attain the services of a personal trainer. We expect you to try to become more active. We want you to pursue exercise, and athletic endeavors safely. That being said, personal trainers are certified professionals and gyms are usually run by dedicated fitness professionals. These people change lives every day and help people achieve their fitness goals. If you have the financial means a gym, personal trainer, or both might be the perfect solution. We have been members of gyms in the past and have had great results. Gyms and trainers require commitment and dedication, but they are not the only option.

The only thing you need to get into better shape is the body you are born with. Hopefully you have some clothes that would be appropriate to work out in, but if you do not, just use what you have. A nice pair of running or walking shoes would be ideal, but if that is not an option for you right now, use what you have. We just want to get you up and moving more than you are now. If you sit in a chair or on the couch all day, we want you to get out in the sun and go for a short walk. When that is easy for you maybe you will want to go for a short walk in the evening after dinner. After a while those short walks will become longer walks and you will be well on your way to fitness, health, and immunity. If you live a more active lifestyle, we want you to push your limits. Those with active careers nd lifestyles need to realize that working is not enough to keep you in shape particularly as you age into your mid 30's and beyond. You have to push your limits. You need to find time for a simple exercise regime, if you can walk, then walk; if you can jog, then jog; if you can run, then run. Getting outside and moving around is so good for your mind, body, and soul. The urge to exercise is a natural progression that is the result of your work on your mind and diet. They all work together wonderfully to raise the level of your health. When you bring your health to a better state, you bring your immunity to a better state.

We told you about an app for smart phones that helps you manage your diet. There are also many free apps that will help you exercise. The incredible thing about these apps is that they connect to myfitnesspal and inform them of the calories you have burned during your workouts. That way you can manage your diet and get a complete picture of what is going on. When it comes to ways to get fit for free the smart phone, tablet, or computer are definitely the best way to do it. These apps are modern technological blessings. There has never been a time before when you could manage your diet, be physically trained, and log all of your activity for free. Smart phones and apps have really made gyms and personal trainers a thing of the past. Why pay money to a gym, and trainer; put money into gas, or public transportation; and take time out of your busy schedule to commute to the work out? Why would we do that when it is all on our phone for free? Maybe the apps are not as good as a personal trainer, but they are free and you have your phone with you wherever you go. With these apps you can do your work out at your level and pace anywhere in the world. You can even complete these exercises in a hotel room or bedroom. Our favorite programs are runkeeper for walking and jogging, and Fitstar for short intense workouts you can do anywhere. We only use the free versions, the free versions of these apps are all you will ever need. They even work with heart rate monitors.

You are now flooding your mind with positive thoughts, improving your diet, exercising more, and tracking it all on your smartphone. The next step in body is Supplementation.

Vitamins and minerals are essential for building your super body. Now that you have started charting everything that you are eating in *My Fitness Pal* or something like it you will find a screen that lists all of your nutritional requirements and FDA recommended daily values. Notice which nutrients you are deficient in, and if you can incorporate those into your diet. If you cannot, supplement deficiencies with vitamins. Purchase the best supplements within your means. It has been our experience that Puritans Pride has excellent value and quality. Let us say here, that no product that we have named specifically is compensating us in any way. We are mentioning actual things that we have used and have found to be helpful. There are other brands, devices, and apps that are just as good if not better. In the world of vitamins, and herbal supplements there are many options. As always you should consult a doctor or a healthcare professional. There are vast amounts of knowledge and opinions on the internet. If you are uninsured, or cannot afford to go to the doctor, supplements and vitamins can be a very helpful preventative measure for overall health and well being. You can get quality herbal supplements on the internet, in pharmacies, grocery stores, organic food stores, and holistic health centers to name a few. Often big chain pharmacies have free clinics where you can consult a healthcare professional. Organic Grocery stores and holistic healing centers often have resident herbalists. From our personal experience these people have been extremely helpful, knowledgeable, and friendly. They are not trying to sell you things you do not need. Most importantly they genuinely care about your health and the health of the whole community. In our neighborhood we are lucky enough to have an holistic pharmacy. These people are the perfect blend of traditional pharmacology and new age holistic healing. They even make custom supplements for you. That way you can have your own customized blend.

4 <u>THE H2O2 PROTOCOL OR THE OXYGEN CLEANSE</u>

Hydrogen peroxide(H2O2) is water (H2O) with an extra atom of oxygen loosely attached to it that plays a vital role in both the health of our planet and the health of our bodies. Oxygen is nature's purifier. Dr. Edward Carl Rosenow was Head of experimental biology for the Mayo foundation from 1914-1944. He published over three hundred medical papers. Thirty-eight of which appeared in the Journal of the American Medical Association. He believed that systemic diseases began in the mouth.[1] *"Dr. Rosenow's investigations consistently demonstrated*

1

the presence of specifically virulent

nonhemolytic streptococci within the oral focus, primarily in or around teeth and/or tonsils (often without visible symptoms of infection) ; these organisms or their derivatives were directly and clearly implicated in a wide range of diseases - from arthritis to schizophrenia and even including disease of "blood- building tissues" The key to the success of Dr. Rosenow's investigations was the use of a laboriously-developed methodology that most significantly correctly mimicked conditions existing within the human body, particularly involving a range of oxygen supply, rather than the customary reliance on strictly "anaerobic" (zero oxygen) or "aerobic" (as in the air) conditions. The manner in which Dr. Rosenow integrated and refined these concepts into an understanding of a wide range of diseases may even come to be recognized as the high point of 20th century medicine, although his legacy is currently obscure or even maligned. Surprisingly, this has occurred despite the association of Dr. Rosenow with some of the most prominent names in American medical history. Early in his career, Dr. Rosenow worked closely with Frank Billings and Charles H. Mayo, both former AMA Presidents and staunch advocates of the concept of oral focal infection as a key factor in systemic disease." had a theory that our bodies should be looked at as the physical world. That it is filled with different eco-systems that various diseases incubate and thrive in. Unhealthy cells and organisms cannot survive in an oxygen rich environment. That is why oxygenating your blood, tissue, and organs is so important. There are many oxygen therapies available ozone, hydrogen peroxide, Hyperbaric chamber, and breathing pure oxygen to name a few.

A proper diet that focuses on alkalizing the blood helps to oxygenate the body. Exercise helps to oxygenate the blood tremendously. The oxygen cleanse is the most affordable, and easiest to do. When added on to mind and body you reach a whole new level of immunity. We have found it extremely safe.

Never use Hydrogen peroxide that comes in a brown bottle from the drugstore or supermarket. It will poison you because of the preservatives. **Only use food grade hydrogen peroxide that comes from a reputable source.** Call the holistic store before you go to make sure they have it. Double check with the herbalist or person in charge to make sure it is food grade H2O2 and find out what percentage it is. If you buy it online make sure it is food grade hydrogen peroxide and double check the percentage you are buying. There is a big difference between food grade 3% and food grade 35%.

Food Grade Hydrogen peroxide is a hazardous material and cannot be sent through the normal mail. If you buy food grade hydrogen peroxide on the internet and they do not charge you for hazardous materials shipping they are not selling the real thing. Always mark your food grade hydrogen peroxide so that you know what percent you are dealing with(important for safety). **Keep all hydrogen peroxide food grade and brown bottle away from children.** Always dilute food grade Hydrogen peroxide before drinking. **Never drink food grade hydrogen peroxide of any strength directly from a bottle.** Never consume food grade hydrogen peroxide in large concentrations. Food grade hydrogen peroxide is powerful, even though it seems pretty harmless, a little dab will do you. When using food grade hydrogen peroxide that is a higher concentration (12% or more) avoid contact with skin. Three percent is fine and is greatly beneficial for the skin. **Never get any type of hydrogen peroxide in the eyes. If this happens flush out with water, and contact a physician.** If concentrated hydrogen peroxide is accidentally consumed (three percent and above) drink massive amounts of water and get to an ER and or call a physician. When you go on the oxygen cleanse you are only putting in small amounts of food grade H2O2 into distilled water. **You always put your food grade H2O2 in with an eye dropper.** You can get eye dropper bottles at the pharmacy, or your organic grocery or holistic healing center. The most reputable companies on the internet almost always give you an eye dropper bottle for every bottle of food grade H2O2 you buy. We are talking about adding a couple drops to an eight ounce glass of distilled water. Even when the cleanse is at its most intense you are only consuming a very dilute amount. A little bit goes a very long way. As we neared the most intense part of the regime we doubled the amount of distilled water as a form of caution. Use distilled water whenever possible. Some people say that chlorinated water makes the H2O2 inert . We have not found that to be true in our personal experiences. **Always consume food grade H2O2 on an empty stomach. Three hours after eating or one hour before eating. The main concern is that if there were harmful bacteria in your food the H2O2 would attack it, you would have a very upset stomach and feel quite nauseous.** If this happens do not induce vomiting, that could cause aspiration of the H2O2 which could could lead to asphyxiation. We have taken it outside the recommended time due to tight schedules and have never experienced problems. We are all individuals and our bodies can react differently, so always use caution. There is a lot of information about this for free, so please do your research and find the food grade hydrogen peroxide protocol that is right for you. Our local organic market only had food grade 12 % H2O2 so we multiplied by three. That makes it the equivalent of 36%. The amounts added are so small however that we found the extra one percent made no difference.

This is the most common H2O2 home remedy. This is the one that is recommended in nearly every book or website. This particular regimen is attributed to Dr. David G. Williams. We have copied this from pure soul organics. A wonderfully informative website that also offers many free downloads on the subject. You find this by typing in H2O2 protocol, or Dr. David G. Williams to your search engine. The site address is 35h2o2.weebly.com. We added the 12% protocol. All of us have different levels of health and fitness this protocol is a general guideline. If you are suffering from serious conditions you may want to proceed as a slower pace. *"Food grade hydrogen peroxide is dispensed from an eyedropper into an eight ounce glass of distilled water. As the dose increases use more distilled water. Do this three times a day on an empty stomach.*

	35 %	*12 %*
Day 1	*3 drops*	*9 drops*
Day2	*4 drops*	*2 drops*
Day3	*5 drops*	*15 drops*
Day4	*6 drops*	*18 drops*
Day5	*7 drops*	*21 drops*
Day6	*8 drops*	*24 drops*
Day7	*9 drops*	*27 drops*
Day8	*10 drops*	*30 drops*
Day9	*12 drops*	*36 drops*
Day10	*14 drops*	*42 drops*
Day11	*16 drops*	*48 drops*
Day 12	*18 drops*	*56 drops*
Day13	*20 drops*	*62 drops*
Day14	*22 drops*	*68 drops*
Day 15	*24 drops*	*72 drops*

Day16   25 drops   75 drops

If you are healthy and doing this to cleanse, to oxygenate your blood, and ultimately protect yourself from disease then it is time to gradually decrease the dosage to a maintenance level.

The H2O2 Protocol

25 drops 1 time a day every other day for 1 week.
25 drops 1 time a day every third day for 2 weeks.
25 drops 1 time a day every fourth day for 3 weeks.

After that decrease dosage to a comfortable level. It only takes a few drops consistently to keep yourself protected. If you were not the perfect picture of health before you started, and you are curing ailments with this protocol then you should stay at the maximum dosage for one to three weeks. After that decrease the dosage to twenty-five drops food grade 35 percent H2O2 two times a day for one to six months."

Once you feel fully healed or you reach six months, drop down to 25 drops one time a day for a week and then gradually reduce the amount to a couple of drops a day or every other day. To protect against things like Ebola and flesh eating bacteria we recommend two drops per day. **This protocol is for adults only.**

As the body is oxygenating and cleansing itself there are times and ways that these toxins leave the body that are not pleasant. Frequent urination, diarrhea, rashes, acne breakouts, exhaustion, flu like symptoms, and mucus in the urine or stool. These symptoms are the Jarvis-Herxheimer reaction and is the effect of endotoxins produced by the death of pathogens and other harmful organisms in the body. This reaction is also simply called a healing crisis. If it is ever too intense for you step back the dosage a day or two and then go forward. The fact that you are experiencing this is proof that it is working. Stay well hydrated and focused on a healthy diet. These symptoms pass fairly quickly and are actually milestones on your journey to complete health. Vitamin E will help your body use more of the oxygen that you have added. Also a probiotic like acidophilus, kefir, or kombucha. will help establish beneficial flora in the lower bowel. This will further increase immunity and boost the body's own production of H2O2. Later in the book we are going to show you other natural ways of establishing this beneficial flora while getting many more benefits for your body and its immune system.

The following list is from an article published by Dr. David G. Williams the same Doctor whose protocol is listed above. We found it on Educate-yourself.org. He states that it is, *"a partial listing of conditions in which H2O2 therapy has been used successfully:Allergies, Headaches, Altitude Sickness, Herpes Simplex, Alzheimer's, Herpes Zoster, Anemia, HIV Infection, Arrhythmia, Influenza, Asthma, Insect Bites, Bacterial Infections, Liver Cirrhosis, Bronchitis, Lupus, Cancer, Multiple Sclerosis, Candida, Parasitic Infections, Cardiovascular Disease, Parkinson's Disease, Chronic Pain, Prostate Issues, Diabetes type II, Rheumatoid Arthritis, Cerebral Vascular disease, Periodontal Disease, Diabetic Gangrene, Shingles, Sinusitis, Digestion Problems, Sore Throat, Epstein-Barr infection, Ulcers, Emphysema, Viral Infections, Food Allergies, Warts, Fungal Infections, Yeast Infections, and gingivitis."*

Dr. David G. Williams claims that all these conditions have been successfully treated with H2O2 therapy. We figured with all this to gain and not much to lose why not give this protocol a try. We are glad we did. At this point we would like to share what our personal experiences were with the oxygen cleanse.

Once we learned about this H2O2 home remedy we thoroughly researched it and weighed out the pros and cons for ourselves, and then decided to do it. The next day we called up our local organic market and asked them if they carried food grade H2O2 . They told us that they did and so we rushed with excitement to buy some. To our disappointment they only had food grade 12% H2O2. We figured that if we multiplied the drops three

times we would be fine. The store also had brown tinted frontier medicine bottles and eyedropper lids for them. We purchased the food grade 12% H2O2, a frontier medicine bottle and an eyedropper lid for the bottle. All said and done less than twenty dollars. We rushed home to start the protocol. We then started day one which would have been three drops of 35% food grade H2O2, but for us it was nine drops of 12% food grade H2O2 in distilled water. First dose no problem. After the last dose that evening we experienced our first Jarvis-Herxheimer reaction(healing crisis) in the form of fatigue and flu like symptoms. It was uncomfortable and made us wonder what we got ourselves into. The next morning however we woke up feeling terrific. The most amazing thing was that we woke up without any pain. We are used to waking up sore because we were still recovering from our workouts, and daily lives from the previous day. That morning was different, no pain of any kind, and actually feeling well rested. Not bad for immediate results. Throughout the rest of the day we felt wonderful. The most prominent thing being deeper stronger breaths than we had taken in years. All this and in just a day or two. As the first week progressed another thing became apparent, we no longer needed Ibuprofen, or any other pain medication to get through our workouts or our active days in general. Joint and muscle pain was something we had accepted as we got older. We always figured take a pill if the pain was to bad and get on with life. Neither of us has had anything but daily vitamin supplements since we started this protocol. The other pills that we stopped taking in the first week were over the counter allergy medications. For us seasonal allergies went away almost overnight. If the only thing this cleanse did was that we would still consider it a success. We also made a three percent food grade H2O2 concentration that we applied to our faces with cotton balls twice a day. Every couple of days we would put a few drops of food grade three percent H2O2 in our ears. Viral and bacterial infections love to hide in the ears. Ears play a big part in our immunity. As we progressed to the second week and higher doses things went splendidly. Cardiovascular wise we felt tremendously stronger and we were able to run farther and faster. We experienced an overall sense of well being and health. Our complexions became amazingly clear and people started to tell each of us that we had glowing complexions. Complete strangers would tell us how healthy we looked. Our resting heart rates had both dropped significantly in the second week. During that second week a good friend came to visit us right after a workout. As we were hanging out he could not believe how healthy we had become. He has known us for years and seen us at different levels of out of shape. He noticed that we had lost weight, gained muscle tone, had a healthy vibrant glow. He even thought that J's hair was growing back and getting thicker. He jokingly referred to the concoction as wolverine juice. It is not named after the fictional superhero, but rather the sinewy beast that lives in the cold north and is feared by everything including bears and humans. That is actually how you start to feel, you feel like nothing can hurt you, no disease or illness can touch you. We have called it that ever since. As we started the third week and neared the maximum dosage we started to feel the healing and cleansing kicking in. Healing crisis became more frequent, but nothing serious. Mainly just a general malaise or fatigue. Some days diarrhea, and quite frequent urination. At times you could just feel the sickness, toxins, and calcification coming out of every pore not to mention every bowel movement. It was at this same time however that we both noticed that the other was not snoring anymore. we know many people, including one of us, who have spent a great deal of money attending sleep studies to deal with sleep apnea and snoring. We also know a great number of people who have spent a great deal of money on contraptions and remedies for snoring. Stopping our snoring alone was worth the twenty dollar start up cost. When we reached the maximum dose we increased the amount of distilled water. We reached the maximum dose without any mishaps. We decided that for the maximum benefit we should go all the way, so we opted to stay on maximum strength for three weeks. That is 25 drops of 35% food grade H_2O_2 in distilled water three times a day. For us it was 75 drops of 12% food grade H_2O_2 three times a day. 75 drops from the dropper is quite a bit. One of the downsides of using 12% food grade H_2O_2 is the number of drops you have to use, it can be quite tedious, but trust us very rewarding. We are not going to lie, the three weeks at maximum strength were very difficult to say the least. We experienced exhaustion, headaches, and irritability in the first week. These symptoms were not constant, they would disappear as quickly as they appeared. One night we would be irritable the next night fine. We noticed that while on the maximum dose our resting heart rates went up, but they were still lower than when we started. The second week of the full dosage was not as hard as the first had been. We still experienced healing crisis, but not as much. A day of diarrhea in the morning, a night of restlessness, or occasional exhaustion, these were the extant of the second week's downside. Something amazing was happening as well. You could feel it working inside you, different places, at different times. It never hurt or was in the least bit painful. It was almost as if you could feel the scrubbing bubbles of oxygen doing their work inside the body. We have to admit when you feel it working in your heart it can be a bit spooky, but so is heart disease. As the second week of full strength came to a close the cleanse became more intense. In the third week of maximum strength the detoxing seemed overwhelming at times. During this process when we experienced the worst healing crisis we still felt better than we did before we started. The benefits that we enjoyed up to this point were nothing short of miraculous, and definitely worth the different forms of healing crises. The downsides of this home remedy were for us at least nothing more than minor annoyances. After the three weeks at maximum strength we stepped down to the maximum dose twice a day. Everything returns to normal fairly quickly; actually at times you miss the third dose. We considered this step a new start for everything. It was a time to make a deeper commitment to our exercise and our diet. It was time to burst forth with health and energy. That week we ordered 35% H2O2 online from WWW.pureh2o2forhealth.com. All said and done one gallon of 35% H2O2 cost us $56.00 after hazardous materials shipping and the discount code. The package arrived within five days. We were both impressed with the speed of shipping and the high quality of the product. It is so much easier to dispense 25 drops as opposed to 75 drops. Once you have the gallon of food grade 35 % you can make 3% solution to kill bad bacteria and pathogens on food, and kitchen counters. We made a large quantity of three percent and filled two spray bottles that we bought from the Dollar Store. Always use plastic spray bottles as H2O2 is an oxidant and will rust metal in a shockingly short time. We use one bottle in the kitchen, and the other for the bathroom. Always use caution when handling 35% H2O2. We have found that it will sting your skin and leave a spot that is pure white no matter your skin tone. This bleaching goes away on light skin in about twenty minutes, on darker skin it can take an hour or two. Neither of us felt endangered at any time because we knew what to expect and now you do as well. You would not believe how many uses we have found for for the food grade three percent H_2O_2 dilution.

Some of the many uses we found
Kitchen counter cleaner/sanitizer
Bathroom cleaner/sanitizer,
Preserving organic dairy products
Vegetable cleaner/sanitizer
Poultry cleaner/sanitizer
Meat cleaner/sanitizer
Oxygen Facial 3%
Mouthwash 3%
Pre and apres shower mist
Sanitize and cleans dishwasher
Floor cleaner
Investing in the food grade 35% H_2O_2 was definitely worth the price. The gallon should almost be a year supply for the two of us.. There have been some instances of Jarvis-Herxheimer reactions, but not many. Any time either of us experiences any such reaction we see it for what it is. We have come to see healing crises as proof that we are still healing past illnesses. Throughout this process even when we felt our worst, we still felt better than we did before we started the cleanse. We know deep in our hearts that we are healthier, and our immune systems are much stronger than they have ever been before. Now that we are well on our way

to completing this journey we know that it was worth it. This therapy has changed our lives for the better. We hope that you decide to join us on this part of the journey because we know that it will change your life as well. You will feel better than you have in a long time and any healing crisis encountered will be worth it. We want to leave you with a few closing thoughts on H2O2. H2O2 is only one of the many oxidative remedies or cures. There are many other treatments available to you. Doctors can inject H2O2 into your system, or treat your blood with ozone and inject it back into your system. These are not medical mainstream practices; however there are doctors out there who specialize in these treatments. There are doctors in the U.S., but they are not easy to find, trust us. There is a lot of information about oxidative therapies and even lists available with doctors who practice these methods in books and for free on the internet. When we tried to contact the listed doctors for our area we found out quite quickly that the information on this list was inaccurate. We kept an open mind however and finally decided to do the oxygen cleanse. We are both very grateful that we did. Oxidative therapy, particularly internal injection of Hydrogen Peroxide is currently very popular in California. California is known for being a health conscious state, especially when it comes to holistic medicine. If you had to breathe the air that they have to breathe you would be very interested in holistic prevention as well. We liken the oxygen cleanse to when we added wheat grass into our lives back in the 1990's when we lived in Los Angeles. Wheat grass and the many benefits obtained from it were on the fringe back then. Now wheat grass is fairly mainstream and helping many people. There are many doctors outside the U.S. Who practice Oxidative therapy. Many Americans have sought out oxidative treatments in Europe and South America, and other parts of the world. If you are suffering from a life threatening disease we urge you to seek out a doctor who practices Ozone or H2O2 therapy. Many claim that the home remedy works amazingly One of these is emphysema. We have heard adding one ounce 35% food grade H2O2 to a gallon of chlorine free water in a vaporizer can help with breathing. We have also heard that internal injections of H2O2 administered by a physician are the best way to go. Research your conditions, ailments, and and be honest with the severity of them. Once you have done that, decide what course of action is best for you. You after all, are the only person in the world who is responsible for your health. So make your decision wisely. We know that the oxygen cleanse is the most important pillar of protection. We sincerely hope that you work on positivity, diet, exercise, and supplementation; They are all very important pillars. They strengthen your body allowing you to attain the most benefit from your oxygen cleanse. If you only change one thing in your life as a result of this book, we both hope that it is the addition of food grade H2O2 to your daily routine. It will raise your level of immunity and protection. So please as a responsible world citizen who wants to be protected, join us on the incredible journey to perfect health by way of the oxygen cleanse.

The world population has reached seven billion souls. That is an enormous amount of people for modern medicine to care for. If ten percent of the world's population did the oxygen cleanse, we would be a much healthier world. There would be less burden on the world's medical systems because minor illness would be a thing of the past.

5 . FERMENTATION

If you would have told a year ago that our counters would be filled with colorful jars of fruits and veggies slowly rotting in water and a little sea salt, we would have thought that you were delusional. It is in fact true, it does exist and it is the 6th Pillar of the program. If we are going to be serious about health we are going to have to be free to talk about our digestive systems and elimination. To paraphrase the Dalai Lama, our highest function is to make excrement. We used to laugh at that little tidbit of wisdom. We did not understand that 85% of our immune system is housed in our digestive system. We always knew that it was an important part of maintaining and achieving overall health, but we did not realize the magnitude of the importance of our guts.

We have learned that the stomach is being looked at by Scientist as a second brain. 90% of the body's Serotonin is produced in the stomach. Serotonin is involved in certain neurological processes including sleep, depression and memory. We really must take stomach health as seriously as we do our mental health because we are learning that they are very dependent on each other. Did you know that your stomach actually sends[2] neurological impulses to your brain? What is it saying? Our guess is, "help me, I'm outnumbered down here there

---

2

http://www.scientificamerican.com/article/gut-second-brain/
Feb 12, 2010 |By Adam Hadhazy

are 100,000 bacteria; please make sure that you are cultivating the beneficial bacteria, that I have a symbiotic relationship with." Thus enters fermented fruits and vegetables. They are superfoods that are packed with probiotics, very tasty, and quite easy to make. Probiotics are of course the good bacteria that promote the growth of the beneficial flora that we need in our bowels. Fermented foods are also thought to be natural chelators, meaning that they help to draw heavy metals out of your body so that they can be eliminated.As with everything else do the best that you can, if you can afford to buy a fermenting crock, or any of the systems that are available for purchase please do so. If you cannot then a glass jar will work just as well. Let your imagination run wild. All that you need is a glass jar, distilled water, a little salt, and whatever fruit or veggies that you have in your fridge. Some people use Whey starters as they can then get a jump start on the fermentation process and save time. We prefer wild fermentation. It is easy, first you clean your vegetables and then cut them however you like; for example, grated, thick chunks, or any texture in between. Mix your ingredients and pack the jar as tightly as you can using hands that are of course very clean. One teaspoon of sea-salt per quart. Fill the jar that you have tightly packed with water, close, and leave on your kitchen counter until ready. Gasses will be produced inside the jars as the lacto-fermentation process is unfolding. Be sure to burp your jars to avoid excess pressure buildup, and moisture seepage. Make sure that water covers all of the food materials. Let stand from anywhere between two to fourteen days. Beware that it is a pungent pastime that you are embarking on, and that broccoli is an egregious offender. You are the judge of when it is done, taste it as you are burping it. That is one of the great things about fermenting you can really experiment. When you have a flavor profile that is acceptable to you simply put the jar in the fridge as that will slow the fermentation process to a crawl. Thereby allowing storage in the refrigerator for a prolonged amount of time. Like any science experiment you will have great success, and at times you will wonder what was I thinking. We once tried a mixture of bok choy,seaweed,and carrots; to be honest that was a little too heavy duty for us. We have found that we really like making sauerkraut using green and red cabbages. We also enjoy fermented radishes, garlic, corn, and cauliflower. Fermented fruit not so much. We tried Apples,Pears, and Cherries and did not really like the saltiness of the fruit. It really is up to you, everyone has a different pallet, do not be afraid to explore and experiment. Below you will find the recipe for a simple beet salad that has become a staple side dish of our dinners and sometimes lunch too. This delicious and healthy recipe is scrumptious.

Beet Salad
Ingredients:
Fermented beets: about a half cup per serving finely chopped
Fermented green cabbage: ½ cup shredded
fermented radishes: 3 per serving coarsely chopped
Fermented Parsnips: ½ cup chopped finely
Fermented Garlic: 2-3 pieces finely chopped
Pickled Mushrooms: ¼ cup chopped
Blue Cheese: at your discretion

In a bowl combine all vegetable ingredients, mix and add in blue cheese. You can add a little balsamic vinegar and oil, or use balsamic salad dressing. We have tried it both ways and have come to the conclusion that it taste great if you use a dressing or if you choose not to.o think of fermented veggies as being a crossword puzzle for our second brain... our stomach. Just like one should exercise the mind one should also exercise the stomach. Do not let it get lazy by consuming easy non-nourishing toxic fast or easy foods prepared in a microwave oven. Connect with what you are putting into your body and fuel it on a deeper more meaningful level. We are eating mindfully, we have learned how to prepare at least one of the right kinds of food that we should be ingesting. That in its own right is very emotionally satisfying. "Heal thyself," starts to make a little more sense. There are many things that we can do for ourselves to make sure that we are performing as optimally as possible and those are the things that we should now be doing. We have to take responsibility for the things that we stuff our faces with. All Fast and Junk foods are loaded with addictive and harmful preservatives and additives. Be strong and forgo those things;

they are poison and punishment foods. We love ourselves enough to prepare and eat life giving true comfort foods.

For well over a millennium the people of Russia,Ukraine and other Slavic states have enjoyed an amazing life affirming beverage that is known as Kvass. Tolstoy felt the need to mention it in not only one but three novels: *Anna Karenina, War and Peace*, and *The Death of Ivan Ilyvich*. Dostoevsky has *Aloysha* the youngest son in *The Brothers Karamazov* living in a monastery that brews their own Kvass. Chekhov has *Lopakhin* the ex-serf that ends up owning the estate mention kvass very early in *The Cherry Orchard*. If three of the greatest literary minds of all time thought enough of kvass to mention it then of course we can give it its own chapter. It is in fact the eighth pillar of our Ebola and all other infectious disease busting manifesto. Made from just beetroot, water and salt. This pillar is just as important as the oxygen cleanse! Beet Kvass is a simple yet potent additive to our wellness arsenal. Beets are a superfood, they have been studied extensively for their medically therapeutic properties. Beets are full of nitrates, which assist in the production of nitric oxide. Nitric oxide widens and relaxes blood vessels which leads to lower blood pressure. This is what WebMD says about nitrates, *"Nitrates also dilate veins throughout the body so that they can hold more blood. This reduces the amount of blood going back to the heart, reducing the heart's workload."*

In 2010 a study was performed at Queen Mary University of London in which it was shown that:
"beetroot and nitrate capsules are equally effective in lowering blood pressure indicating that it is the nitrate content of beetroot juice that underlies its potential to reduce blood pressure. We also found that only a small amount of juice is needed – just 250ml - to have this effect, and that the higher the blood pressure at the start of the study the greater the decrease caused by the nitrate." The

above quoted article was published in the American Heart Association online journal Hypertension.

Beet Kvass is used in cancer therapy throughout Europe and is frequently recommended to cancer patients undergoing radiation therapy . Beet Kvass is also a good source of natural iodine. Iodine is an essential trace element. The Encyclopedia Britannica defines a trace element as follows:

*"a **trace element,** also called Micro nutrient, in biology, any chemical element required by living organisms in minute amounts, usually as part of a vital enzyme, a cell-produced catalytic protein. Exact needs vary among species, but commonly required plant micronutrients include copper, boron, zinc, manganese, and molybdenum. Animals also require manganese, iodine, and cobalt. Lack of a necessary plant micronutrient in the soil causes plant deficiency diseases; lack of animal micronutrients in the soil may not harm the plants, but, without them, animals feeding solely on those plants develop deficiency diseases."*

Beets are also packed full of Potassium, Magnesium, and many other vital nutrients. They also have Betacyanin Which has been shown in studies to slow cancerous growths in prostate and breast cancer cells.

Easy Beet Kavass

Fill the largest glass jar that you own half full with beets that have been scrubbed and peeled and chopped coarsely. We use a gallon glass jar that has a pour spout. Add a teaspoon of sea salt, or rock salt. Do not use iodized table salt. Fill the container with distilled water. Cover the top of jar, set on counter two- fourteen

days. As with all fermentation you are the judge of when your Kvass is done. When it is, strain the contents into another glass container. Be sure to scoop out the white mold that will form on the surface. White mold is good it is actually the beneficial probiotics that we are looking for. If you notice black mold forming in the Kvass throw it out. As with all fermented foods brown or black mold is not to be ingested the foods are contaminated and have to be thrown out. Trial and error has taught us to remove any beets that start to float in the liquid. We have read that the beets can be reused to make another batch but we have not had much success with that method. We use fresh beets for every new batch of Kvass. Keep in mind that the flavor of your beverage will mellow out in the refrigerator. Kvass is a beautiful, salty, sour drink. We always save the used beets in another jar in the fridge they are great to have around and they have a ton of uses.

The first time that we had Kvass we stared at our wine glasses that held six ounces of beet blood red liquid that was vaguely effervescent. In that moment the myth of the Vampire made perfect sense. It looks like blood with its velvety deep purple hue. The saltiness of it is reminiscent of blood as well. The people who drank it all the time probably looked great for their ages and lived for a very long time. Yeah, sounds like vampires to me. Our little joke as we sip our Kvass these days is that one will look at the other and put on the worst Dracula accent that you can imagine and ask "Do you want to live forever...? Drink Kvass." You feel how good it actually is for you, one has the sensation that the body is actually saying "Thank You" as you finish your glass.

6 OTOLARYNGOLOGICAL HEALTH "EAR NOSE AND THROAT CLEANSE"

The fifth pillar of protection is the Sinus and oral cleanse. The otolaryngological system plays a vital role in your immune system. The free online Oxford English dictionary defines otolaryngology as: *"The branch of medical science that deals with the ear nose and throat."* The ear, nose, and throat work together in harmony to protect us from pathogens, virus, bacteria, and other toxins. Even though Ebola is not an airborne virus, it has the ability to survive on surfaces. Contact with such surfaces could compromise the otolaryngological system. There are many other airborne viruses and bacteria that we are exposed to everyday; these could compromise our immune system right when we need it the most.

The amount of pollutants and toxins in the air today torment our immune systems. We as a world population are experiencing a great many allergies. People have always suffered allergies of one form or another. When you combine the modern diet with the current state of air quality in the world we are creating a recipe for disaster. How many people do you know who suffer from severe allergies? We are fairly sure that if you yourself do not have any allergies, that you at least know a couple people who do suffer them. Medical treatment from allergists and otolaryngologists will provide relief from allergies. Sinus and oral cleanses are beneficial for not only relief of allergic symptoms, but your overall health and immunity as well.

Nasal irrigation is also known as nasal lavage. It is the practice of flushing away excess mucus and debris from the sinus cavity and nose. There are many ways to cleanse or rinse the sinus, the one that we prefer is the Neti Pot. People have been using Neti Pots for millennia . It is one of the most tried and true home therapies available; therefore half of the seventh pillar of protection is the Neti Pot. The Neti Pot is very affordable and extremely safe when used properly. This is a home remedy that we have been using for about a decade now. We first heard of the Neti Pot about a decade prior to that. We had severe head colds and figured what could we lose, so we bought a Neti Pot along with all the other usual over the counter cold remedies. We were both impressed by the Neti Pot from the first use. We were convinced and still are to this day that the Neti Pot helps you rid your body of infection. Many colds and other infections have either been prevented or treated with the Neti Pot by us over the years. Neither of us has missed a day of work due to sickness in three years. Any time either of us has experienced even the slightest tickle in our throat or soft palate we turn to the Neti Pot immediately. The times when we have waited till the day after the symptoms appeared we have fallen ill. The times when we used the Neti Pot at the first sign of illness we have either averted infection or greatly reduced the time for recovery. We believe in the Neti Pot and consider it one of our most important weapons in our health arsenal. You need to use caution and follow the directions, but once you get comfortable with it, we are sure that you are going to love it.

Neti Pots are fairly new to Western culture. The benefits of this home therapy have only been known in the West for about a hundred years. In the east however the Neti Pot has been used since ancient times. The benefits of the Neti Pot have been known for many millennia in India. The discipline of yoga considers Neti Pot an essential tool for physical well being and spiritual enlightenment.

The first recorded use of the Neti Pot is in the ancient Hindu practice of Ayurveda. Neti translates to nasal irrigation in the language Sanskrit. It is believed that the Sanskrit language may have been spoken in India as early as the second millennium BCE. Scholars believe that the language migrated from the region around modern day Iran. The language was spoken long before it arrived in the region which is modern day India and Pakistan. People have been using the Neti Pot for a very long time. Hatha yoga employs the Neti Pot as part of the shatkarma, which is also known as as yogic body cleansing. The use of the Neti Pot is known as Jala Neti in hatha yoga. It is believed that clear nasal passages lead to clear thinking. The Neti Pot became more popular in the west during the late sixties and early seventies. People who went to seek enlightenment in India amongst the great Yogis brought the Neti Pot home with them. Slowly they grew in popularity and were considered a wonderful homeopathic practice. Neti Pots became mainstream in the U.S. when Dr. Oz featured them on *Oprah.*

You can obtain a Neti Pot at almost any pharmacy or drugstore. They are also for sale online. Manufacturers include very important instructions, read them carefully. Neti Pots come in many shapes, sizes and colors. The most popular design looks like a cross between a miniature watering can and a magic lamp containing a genie. The only forms of magic associated with the Neti Pot are its cleansing and healing properties. There are many benefits associated with the Neti Pot. The flushing of bacteria and dirt laden mucus from the nose. It helps with ear infections, and tinnitus. It can help alleviate asthma and bronchitis by clearing the nasal passageways. The Neti Pot is beneficial for eye health; it improves vision while clearing and brightening the eyes. It may help calm and soothe the brain and could help headaches, migraines, and even possibly epilepsy. The Neti Pot improves the senses of taste and smell. It can benefit the pituitary gland and balance hormones. It is believed by many that the Neti Pot brings clarity of mind, increases visualization, and improves meditation. This could definitely help all of us with the first pillar of positive mind. It is even thought by some that it could help moderate mood and behavioral disorders. We can both attest to the Neti Pot's effectiveness.

There are some risks with the Neti Pot, but those are nullified with responsible use. The FDA has issued a warning concerning Neti Pots. The warning states that improper use of Neti Pots could result in serious and even potentially fatal infections. The main safety precaution is the use of sterile water for the nasal rinse. Never use tap water, it could be harmful or fatal. Municipal tap water can have small amounts of bacteria, microorganisms, and protozoa. They are supposedly harmless to swallow. They could be potentially lethal in the nasal passages, because they could remain alive and cause serious illness. The whole point of this book is prevent illness, so please use distilled water, the purest sodium chloride available(never use iodized salt), and sterilize your neti pot with food grade H2O2 or food grade grain alcohol(Everclear). Always rinse and dry after sterilization. Never use iodized salt. Burning your nasal passage and sinus is a potential problem associated with improper Neti Pot use. You want to use warm water, but if the water is too hot it could scald or burn you inside your nasal passage. That would be disastrous, so please use warm distilled water for your safety. Cool or cold water is also uncomfortable, but it will not injure you like hot water. We have experienced water that was just a little too hot. Neither of us were injured, but it was far from comfortable. We experienced fairly intense pain and profuse watering from the eyes. Trust us, better to be lukewarm and safe than have scalding water run through the inside of your head. We advise you to follow the manufacturers instruction and heed the FDA warning about tap water. Through proper use the cleansing and healing that takes place is wondrous.

Here is our personal guide for Neti Pot use. There are two ways to use the Neti Pot:
The first is the method most people use, where you pour the warm distilled saline water solution in one nostril and let it flow through the other nostril. This is the easy way that anyone can do and eventually become comfortable with.

The second way is a technique used by yogis. This is where you pour the water into your nostril and let it flow through your soft palate and out your mouth. It is uncomfortable at first, and can be quite hard to perform. The benefits however are better than the aforementioned method. The first method is quite easy. Use lukewarm to warm distilled water, and a little unprocessed pure organic salt (never use iodized salt). Never use water that is too warm, it could damage the soft tissues of the nasal passages. Salinity depends on personal preference, we advise you to start with a fairly low salt level and work your way up to the salinity level that you prefer. Mix the solution very well, make sure that all the salt has dissolved and is not sitting on the bottom of your Neti Pot. We usually stir briskly reversing direction at irregular intervals. Lean over your bathroom sink and tilt your head to the right, less than ninety degrees, but almost there. Pour the warm distilled saline solution into your left nostril and let it flow out of your right nostril into the sink. Gently blow both nostrils into the sink basin. After that blow your nose gently into a tissue a couple of times. Repeat the entire process on the other side. Always clean and sterilize/sanitize the sink when you are finished. Always clean, sterilize/sanitize, and completely dry your Neti Pot after each use, so it is ready for the next use.

The second method is the one that is in use by Yogis. It is more complex and difficult to fully master. Never do this one while you are alone. Always have someone spot you in case you start to choke or asphyxiate. Just getting a little water through the soft palate could have tremendous benefits. Mix the same lukewarm distilled saline solution (never use iodized salt). Mix just like the first time, about 50 brisk stirs reversing direction every once in a while. This time you are going to tilt your head back so that you are looking up at the ceiling. Close your right nostril with your right index finger. Gently insert the Neti Pot spout in your left nostril with your left hand. Relax and see if the water will naturally flow down through your soft palate and into your mouth. If this does not happen naturally we suggest giving a couple gentle snorts. Once you feel water entering your mouth lean forward and spit it out into the sink. Be careful not to aspirate the water as that could cause asphyxiation. If some solution does go down your throat or the wrong pipe, cough it up immediately. The chance of this happening is why we say always have someone there to help you in case you need it. They need to be watching you, because if you do start to choke you might not be able to communicate verbally with your spotter. Once you are satisfied that the first nostril is done it is time to repeat this whole process on the other side.

Since starting the Oxygen Cleanse we have experimented with putting food grade hydrogen peroxide in our Neti Pot. A little food grade hydrogen peroxide goes a long way. From our experience one drop of food grade 35% H_2O_2 is quite adequate. If you are using food grade 12% H_2O_2 we recommend no more than two drops. These recommendations are based on our own experiences with different amounts of drops and different percentages. A little food grade three percent H_2O_2 is probably the safest way to go. There is debate over H_2O_2 in the nasal passageways. Some people believe it is wonderful, while others believe it could be detrimental. We do not put Food Grade H_2O_2 in every time we use the Neti Pot. We add a drop very sparingly every once in a while. We have never experienced ill side effects. What we are comfortable with and works for us, might not be the right option for you. You know yourself and what you can handle better than anyone else. T hat is the first half of the fifth pillar, next is the Oral Cleanse. The Oral Cleanse is the simplest of all the methods discussed in this book. It will cleanse bacteria, toxins, and viruses out of your throat while making your gums healthy, your teeth white, and breath fresh. It will also clear out the harmful streptococci from the mouth and tonsil area. Remember Dr. Rosenow and his discoveries that harmful streptococci in the oral cavity are the cause of mental disorders, arthritis, along with a myriad of other conditions. He identified 35 different forms of streptococci that live in our oral cavity. Let us gargle them away. It is similar to a salt water rinse and gargle, except that it is a food grade three percent or less H_2O_2 rinse and gargle. If you wanted you could add unprocessed, iodine free natural salt, but it is not necessary. Never swallow food grade three percent or more H_2O_2. If you do swallow food grade three percent H_2O_2 by accident drink copious amounts of water and contact a medical professional. As a rule treat it just like any other mouthwash, you would not want to drink that either. After flossing, but before brushing take a small amount of Food grade three percent or less H_2O_2 into your mouth just like normal mouthwash. Swish it around in your mouth over your teeth and gums. Then tilt your head back and gargle for a good long time. Spit about half the liquid out and repeat the process with the remaining half. You will notice that it foams up. That is because the H_2O_2 has been activated in the process of sanitizing your oral cavity. Spit everything out and then rinse and gargle with regular water. The chlorine in tap water will deactivate the H_2O_2 in the oral cleanse.

The FDA approves the use of Brown bottle three percent H_2O_2 as an oral debriding agent. We believe that food grade

H2O2 is a much safer option. Brown bottle, while approved by the FDA for this purpose, contains preservatives and chemicals that can be extremely harmful to you. Food grade three percent H2O2 is a superior option.

So now you are working on positive mindfulness, the body, drinking wolverine juice, eating fermented veggies, and cleansing your otolaryngological system. Your immune system has become quite strong. Aside from that you have also become quite strong Mentally, emotionally, physically, and spiritually. You will notice that you are less prone to depression, and that you are ready for any challenge that life can throw at you.

7 **PUTTING IT ALL TOGETHER**

Now that you have been introduced to the eight pillars of protection. The next step is to put them all into practice. This can be overwhelming, daunting and challenging to say the least. This book proposes a complete overhaul of your life style, this is not easy to implement. The chapters have revealed the steps to ultimate health and superior immunity, but only you can make the commitment to transform yourself. As humans we make commitments and break them constantly. We break commitments to others and worst of all we break commitments to ourselves. The obligations of life can often get in the way of commitments we have made to others or ourselves. When someone breaks a commitment to you it can be very disappointing, we all have experienced this a time or two in our lives. We have to learn to forgive people who break commitments to us and be empathetic to their situation. It can be even more disappointing when we break commitments to ourselves. We all have to learn to forgive ourselves when we break commitments to ourselves as well. On any great journey there will be times when the path is treacherous and you fall down in a moment of weakness. Forgive yourself and move on and pursue that commitment with even more passion when you start again. Try your best, when you fail, forgive yourself and move on. No matter how many times you fail repeat this process and you will reap the benefits of all the five pillars of protection.

There is only one pillar that we urge you not to start and stop. That is the oxygen cleanse. If you make a commitment to the full cure you have to stick with it until it is done. The benefits of committing to the complete cure are nothing short of miraculous. There are currently thousands of people on this same protocol right now. There are currently thousands who are learning about it and considering it. Many of them are afraid to make the commitment, or are still undecided. There have been multitudes of people who have committed to this protocol or something like it over the past hundred years or so. There are many testimonials from these people praising food grade H2O2 and they consider it to be the ultimate miracle cure. It is a very difficult choice to make. Do you believe the people who praise this remedy or do you believe the people who say it could be harmful. Only you can make that choice and then commit. Once you do commit please stick with it. If you miss a dose here or there that is fine. Do not miss multiple days. Starting and stopping this regimen could greatly reduce all the benefits that could be realized by completing the entire course. Those benefits are healing past sickness, and preventing future illness and disease. Nothing in life is one hundred percent so give the oxygen cleanse the best chance it can have by completing the protocol. It is a seven month commitment to complete the full cleanse. Once you have completed it, you should never have to do it again. You can stay on a minimal dose to stay oxygenated, but you will never have to do it with such intensity ever again.

Do the best you can with all the other pillars. We know that no one is perfect. There will be times when you miss workouts. There will be times when your meals lack nourishment. Sometimes you will give in to cravings. There will definitely be times when your mind and attitude will not be as positive as you would have hoped. As for supplements of course you will forget to take them at some point. All these things are understandable and completely fine. No one expects you to do the Neti Pot everyday. Do the best you can do to implement all these pillars into your life. Once you see how fara little effort goes with each of these pillars you will be amazed how much better your whole life has become. Once you start realizing the benefits of the five pillars, you are going to want to make a deeper commitment to them as well as your overall health in general.

The basic premise is to start to control your mind in a positive way. The power of the mind and subconscious alone can completely protect you from all sickness and disease. It takes a great deal of work to master. It can take an entire lifetime to master the power of positivity. Then you start to work on your diet and develop healthy eating habits. At this point you start to add light exercise into your routine. After that you add supplements into your life. These two pillars are the foundation of the program. Do the best you can with all of them. Once you have a strong foundation then you begin to incorporate the other three pillars of protection to the best of your ability.

This book is concerned with improving your life. We want you to be healthier than you are right now. We know that human habits are hard to break and that our vices can be impossible to give up. Nowhere in this book have we asked anyone to stop smoking, drinking, or any other harmful habits. You already know that these actions are bad for you. There is nothing we can do or say to make you stop them, only you can do that. We want you to be mentally, spiritually, and physically as strong as you can be. Once you start to see the transformation in your life we hope that you gain the strength to address your vices.

We wish you all the success possible with this program. We know once this program has become a part of your life you will be a happier, healthier person. Once you have reaped the rewards of this program we hope that you can share it with other people. It is said that there are only six degrees of separation between all of humanity. When you start to experience the miracles that this program can produce, we ask you to share it with six people that are important to you. If we can all do this we can produce a mass wave of healing power across the world. The results will be astounding. We both dream of a happy, healthy world, where every human can achieve their dream in safety and peace. We know that getting as many people as possible on this program would be a good start to realizing our dream. Please join us on our crusade   for   ultimate   health   and   happiness.

ABOUT THE AUTHORS

J. Guinan Stevens and C.L. Carmen live in Maryland with their two cats. They have previously authored the "Ebola Survival Kit" which is also available on Amazon and kindle direct download.